Current Medications & Supplements

Start Date	Medication/Supplement	Dosage	Frequency

Allergies & Sensitivities _______________________________

New Protocol & Observation Notes "Introducing a new medication or supplement is a process, not an event. Use this space to document start dates and how your body responds during the transition. Your data is the bridge between a 'side effect' and a breakthrough.

____

____

____

____

My 90-Day Health Commitment

Journey Start Date: ___________   Starting Weight: ___________

90-Day Milestone Date: ___________   Goal Weight / Outcome: ___________

Weekly Workout Goal: _____________ Days

Cycle Goal: ____

Insulin Strategy: ____

Primary Symptom Focus: ______________________________________

Use this space to write a detailed commitment to yourself. Why are you starting this now? What does "showing up" look like for you on the hard days?

____

____

____

____

Signature: _____________________

Date: _________

By Angela Hayes

THE PCOS
PROTOCOL

Mapping the 150+ Connection: A 90-Day
Biometric & Symptom Tracker

By Angela Hayes

The 150+ Connection

A Note from Angela....

Did you know there are over 150 conditions and symptoms connected to PCOS?

For years, I felt like my body was a series of random glitches. I had my PCOS diagnosis, but then came the Weight Gain, the GERD, the Vitiligo, and the Dry Eyes. I was frustrated because I didn't see the connection. I thought I just had a 'bad' deck of health cards.

I didn't realize that my body wasn't failing; it was signaling. On the next few pages, you will find a Medical Blueprint of our core conditions, followed by the rest of the 150+ signals that make up this complex map. These pages are designed to help you bring a full, undeniable report of your health to your medical team.

Angela Hayes

Hey Sis, Let's Take Our Strength Back.

I was diagnosed with PCOS at 23. Like many of you, I spent years feeling like my body was a mystery I couldn't solve. I've seen the scale hit 265 lbs, and I've battled the physical and mental toll of HS (Hidradenitis Suppurativa) and Hirsutism.

I didn't create this logbook because I have all the answers—I created it because I needed a better way to track the data. As a website designer and entrepreneur, I know that what gets measured gets managed. This isn't just a journal; it's your personal biometric dashboard.

Whether you are navigating IVF, managing insulin resistance, or just trying to find your way back to yourself, you are not alone in this fight. Use these pages to be radically honest with yourself and to bring clear, undeniable data to your medical team.

Your journey is yours to own. Let's get to work.

Angela Hayes
Founder of Aivonax

My Medical Blueprint

☐ PCOS (Polycystic Ovary Syndrome)   Date: _______________

☐ Weight Gain / Weight Fluctuations   Date: _______________

☐ Hirsutism (Excess hair growth)   Date: _______________

☐ HS (Hidradenitis Suppurativa)   Date: _______________

☐ Infertility / Irregular Cycles   Date: _______________

☐ Type 2 Diabetes   Date: _______________

☐ Insulin Resistance / Prediabetes   Date: _______________

☐ NAFLD (Fatty Liver Disease)   Date: _______________

☐ Hypertension (High Blood Pressure)   Date: _______________

☐ High Cholesterol   Date: _______________

☐ Hormonal Acne (Cystic/Jawline)   Date: _______________

☐ Obstructive Sleep Apnea   Date: _______________

☐ Memory Loss / "Brain Fog   Date: _______________

☐ Anxiety / Depression   Date: _______________

☐ Chronic Fatigue   Date: _______________

Digestive & Metabolic

[ ] GERD / Acid Reflux
[ ] IBS / Chronic Bloating
[ ] Chronic Constipation
[ ] Food Sensitivities
[ ] Excessive Thirst
[ ] Sugar "Crashes" (Shakiness)
[ ] Gallbladder Sludge/Issues
[ ] Slow Digestion
[ ] Metallic Taste in Mouth
[ ] Intense Salt Cravings
[ ] Nausea when Fasting
[ ] "Heavy" Stomach Feeling
[ ] Heartburn after Water
[ ] Frequent Burping
[ ] Sudden Food Aversions

Eyes, Ears & Sensory

[ ] Dry Eye Syndrome
[ ] Blurred Vision (Intermittent)
[ ] Sensitivity to Light
[ ] Tinnitus (Ringing in Ears)
[ ] Ear Wax Buildup (Excessive)
[ ] Vertigo / Dizziness
[ ] Eye Twitching
[ ] Sensory Overload (Noise/Lights)
[ ] Pressure Behind Eyes
[ ] Floaters in Vision
[ ] Poor Night Vision
[ ] Red/Bloodshot Eyes
[ ] Itchy Ear Canals

Skin, Hair & Nails

[ ] Vitiligo
[ ] Skin Tags (Neck/Armpits)
[ ] Keratosis Pilaris (Chicken Skin)
[ ] Oily Scalp / Dandruff
[ ] Brittle / Ridged Nails
[ ] Easy Bruising
[ ] Slow Wound Healing
[ ] Cracked Heels
[ ] Eczema / Psoriasis Flare-ups
[ ] Hives / Unexplained Rashes
[ ] Skin Sensitivity to Touch
[ ] Thinning Eyebrows (Outer edge)
[ ] Pale Skin / Anemia signs
[ ] Excessive Sweating (Hyperhidrosis)
[ ] Body Odor

Brain, Mood & Sleep

[ ] Panic Attacks
[ ] Night Terrors / Vivid Dreams
[ ] Insomnia (Difficulty falling asleep)
[ ] Early Waking (3 AM Wake-ups)
[ ] "Wired but Tired" Feeling
[ ] ADHD / Focus Issues
[ ] Irritability (PCOS "Rage")
[ ] Seasonal Affective Disorder
[ ] Depersonalization
[ ] Decision Fatigue
[ ] Restless Leg Syndrome
[ ] Sleep Paralysis

Joint, Muscle & Body Pain

[ ] Pelvic Pain / Heaviness
[ ] Lower Back Pain
[ ] Joint Stiffness (Morning)
[ ] Muscle Weakness
[ ] Clicking/Popping Joints
[ ] Plantar Fasciitis (Heel Pain)
[ ] Carpal Tunnel Symptoms
[ ] Neck Tension / Stiffness
[ ] "Growing Pains" in Legs
[ ] Tailbone Tenderness
[ ] Random Nerve "Zaps"
[ ] Costochondritis (Chest wall pain)
[ ] Fibromyalgia Signs
[ ] Sharp Ovulation Pain (Mittelschmerz)

Inflammatory & Systemic

[ ] Chronic Sinus Congestion
[ ] Frequent Colds / Weak Immunity
[ ] Night Sweats
[ ] Heart Palpitations
[ ] Swollen Ankles (Edema)
[ ] Cold Hands & Feet
[ ] Temperature Intolerance
[ ] Bleeding Gums
[ ] Recurrent Mouth Ulcers
[ ] Swollen Lymph Nodes
[ ] Shortness of Breath (Mild)
[ ] Frequent Urination
[ ] Recurrent Yeast Infections / UTIs
[ ] Allergic Shiners (Under-eye circles)
[ ] Heavy Limb Feeling

Neurological & Respiratory

[ ] Hand Tremors
[ ] Dizziness when Standing (POTS-like)
[ ] Poor Physical Coordination
[ ] Numbness/Tingling in Extremities
[ ] Chronic Cough (Non-illness)
[ ] Shallow Breathing
[ ] Sleep Hypoventilation
[ ] Morning Headaches
[ ] Feeling "Air Hungry"
[ ] Post-nasal Drip
[ ] Excessive Phlegm

Dental & Oral Health

[ ] Chronic Dry Mouth
[ ] Recurrent Canker Sores
[ ] Sensitive Teeth
[ ] Gum Inflammation / Swelling
[ ] Recurrent Oral Thrush
[ ] Grinding Teeth (Bruxism)
[ ] Jaw Tension / TMJ Pain
[ ] Coated Tongue
[ ] Halitosis (Persistent Bad Breath)

Reproductive & Sexual Health

[ ] Severe PMS / PMDD
[ ] Mid-cycle Spotting
[ ] Low Libido (Sex Drive)
[ ] Vaginal Dryness
[ ] Ovarian Cyst Pain (Rupture history)
[ ] Pain during Intercourse
[ ] Recurrent Bacterial Vaginosis (BV)
[ ] Tender Breasts (Cyclical)

Psychological & Emotional

[ ] Intrusive Thoughts
[ ] Rejection Sensitivity
[ ] Overthinking / Rumination
[ ] Low Self-Esteem
[ ] Mood "Crashes" after Meals
[ ] Emotional Eating
[ ] Social Withdrawal
[ ] Feelings of Worthlessness
[ ] Heightened Stress Response

More Digestive & Metabolic

[ ] Constant Hunger (Polyphagia)
[ ] Sudden "Hangry" Episodes
[ ] Intense Sweet Cravings
[ ] Loose Stools / Diarrhea
[ ] Feeling Full after Small Bites
[ ] Upper Abdominal Tenderness
[ ] Foul-smelling Gas
[ ] Difficulty Swallowing (Globus)
[ ] Sulfur Burps

General & Miscellaneous

[ ] Heightened Startle Response
[ ] Chronic Low Vitamin D
[ ] Chronic Low Iron / Ferritin
[ ] Sensitivity to Chemical Smells
[ ] Swollen Fingernails (Clubbing)
[ ] Vertical Ridges on Nails
[ ] White Spots on Nails (Zinc deficiency)
[ ] Pale Tongue / Gums
[ ] Slow Reflexes
[ ] General Malaise ("Feeling Sickish")
[ ] Recurring Low-grade Fever

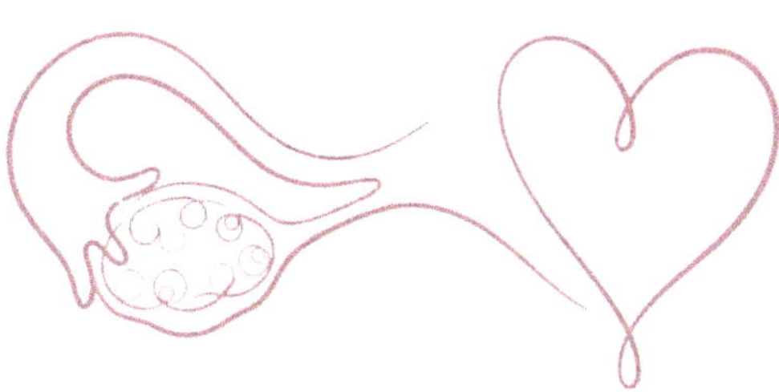

Custom Medical Blueprint & Care Team

Personal Diagnoses & Health Concerns

Use this table for any additional conditions or specific concerns not listed on the previous page.

Condition / Diagnosis	Date

Notes / Status

____

____

____

____

My Specialist Directory

Keep your care team's details in one place for easy reference during emergencies or referrals.

Endocrinologist: _______________________________________

OBGYN / Fertility Specialist: _______________________________

Dermatologist (HS/Acne Care): _______________________________

PCP / Internal Medicine: _______________________________

Daily Vitality Log

The Morning Baseline

Date: _____/______/________   Date of Cycle: _____/______/________

Blood Pressure: _____ / _____

Waking Glucose: ___________   Weight: ____________

The PCOS Cycle Tracker

Flow: [ ] Light   [ ] Med   [ ] Heavy   [ ] Spotting

Ovulation Test: [ ] Positive   [ ] Negative

Cervical Fluid Type: _________   Basal Body Temp: ________

Grooming Log

[ ] Shave   [ ] Wax   [ ] Thread   [ ] Laser

Intensity Scale: 1   2   3   4   5

Daily Habits & Triggers

Movement Goal: [ ] Done!

Mood: 1   2   3   4   5   Energy: 1   2   3   4   5

Caffeine: Alcohol:

The Evidence (150+ Connection)

Symptoms Noticed: ____

Food/Supplements: ____

Daily Vitality Log

The Morning Baseline

Date: _____/_____/_______   Date of Cycle: _____/_____/________

♥ Blood Pressure: ____ / ____

Waking Glucose: __________   Weight: ___________

The PCOS Cycle Tracker

Flow: [ ] Light   [ ] Med   [ ] Heavy   [ ] Spotting

Ovulation Test: [ ] Positive   [ ] Negative

Cervical Fluid Type: ________   Basal Body Temp: _______

Grooming Log

[ ] Shave   [ ] Wax   [ ] Thread   [ ] Laser

Intensity Scale: 1   2   3   4   5

Daily Habits & Triggers

Movement Goal: [ ] Done!

Mood: 1   2   3   4   5   Energy: 1   2   3   4   5

Caffeine: Alcohol:

The Evidence (150+ Connection)

Symptoms Noticed: ____

Food/Supplements: ____

Daily Vitality Log

The Morning Baseline

Date: _____/_____/______   Date of Cycle: _____/_____/________

Blood Pressure: ____ / ____

Waking Glucose: __________   Weight: ___________

The PCOS Cycle Tracker

Flow: [ ] Light   [ ] Med   [ ] Heavy   [ ] Spotting

Ovulation Test: [ ] Positive   [ ] Negative

Cervical Fluid Type: ________   Basal Body Temp: _______

Grooming Log

[ ] Shave   [ ] Wax   [ ] Thread   [ ] Laser

Intensity Scale: 1   2   3   4   5

Daily Habits & Triggers

Movement Goal: [ ] Done!

Mood: 1   2   3   4   5   Energy: 1   2   3   4   5

Caffeine: Alcohol:

The Evidence (150+ Connection)

Symptoms Noticed: ____

Food/Supplements: ____

Daily Vitality Log

The Morning Baseline

Date: ______/______/________   Date of Cycle: ______/______/________

Blood Pressure: _____ / _____

Waking Glucose: ___________   Weight: ____________

The PCOS Cycle Tracker

Flow: [] Light   [] Med   [] Heavy   [] Spotting

Ovulation Test: [] Positive   [] Negative

Cervical Fluid Type: __________   Basal Body Temp: ________

Grooming Log

[] Shave   [] Wax   [] Thread   [] Laser

Intensity Scale: 1   2   3   4   5

Daily Habits & Triggers

Movement Goal: [] Done!

Mood: 1   2   3   4   5   Energy: 1   2   3   4   5

Caffeine: Alcohol:

The Evidence (150+ Connection)

Symptoms Noticed: ____

Food/Supplements: ____

Daily Vitality Log

The Morning Baseline

Date: _____/_____/_______   Date of Cycle: _____/_____/_______

Blood Pressure: _____/_____

Waking Glucose: __________   Weight: ___________

The PCOS Cycle Tracker

Flow: [ ] Light   [ ] Med   [ ] Heavy   [ ] Spotting

Ovulation Test: [ ] Positive   [ ] Negative

Cervical Fluid Type: _________   Basal Body Temp: ________

Grooming Log

[ ] Shave   [ ] Wax   [ ] Thread   [ ] Laser

Intensity Scale: 1   2   3   4   5

Daily Habits & Triggers

Movement Goal: [ ] Done!

Mood: 1   2   3   4   5   Energy: 1   2   3   4   5

Caffeine: Alcohol:

The Evidence (150+ Connection)

Symptoms Noticed: ____

Food/Supplements: ____

Daily Vitality Log

The Morning Baseline

Date: _____/_____/_______   Date of Cycle: _____/_____/_______

Blood Pressure: ____ / ____

Waking Glucose: __________   Weight: ___________

The PCOS Cycle Tracker

Flow: [ ] Light   [ ] Med   [ ] Heavy   [ ] Spotting

Ovulation Test: [ ] Positive   [ ] Negative

Cervical Fluid Type: ________   Basal Body Temp: ________

Grooming Log

[ ] Shave   [ ] Wax   [ ] Thread   [ ] Laser

Intensity Scale: 1   2   3   4   5

Daily Habits & Triggers

Movement Goal: [ ] Done!

Mood: 1   2   3   4   5   Energy: 1   2   3   4   5

Caffeine: ☕ ☕ ☕   Alcohol: 🍷 🍷 🍷

The Evidence (150+ Connection)

Symptoms Noticed: ____

Food/Supplements: ____

Daily Vitality Log

The Morning Baseline

Date: _____/______/________   Date of Cycle: ______/______/_________

Blood Pressure: _____ / _____

Waking Glucose: __________   Weight: ____________

The PCOS Cycle Tracker

Flow: [ ] Light   [ ] Med   [ ] Heavy   [ ] Spotting

Ovulation Test: [ ] Positive   [ ] Negative

Cervical Fluid Type: _________   Basal Body Temp: ________

Grooming Log

[ ] Shave   [ ] Wax   [ ] Thread   [ ] Laser

Intensity Scale: 1   2   3   4   5

Daily Habits & Triggers

Movement Goal: [ ] Done!

Mood: 1   2   3   4   5   Energy: 1   2   3   4   5

Caffeine: Alcohol:

The Evidence (150+ Connection)

Symptoms Noticed: ____

Food/Supplements: ____

Daily Vitality Log

The Morning Baseline

Date: _____/_____/_______   Date of Cycle: _____/______/________

Blood Pressure: ____ / ____

Waking Glucose: __________   Weight: ___________

The PCOS Cycle Tracker

Flow: [ ] Light   [ ] Med   [ ] Heavy   [ ] Spotting

Ovulation Test: [ ] Positive   [ ] Negative

Cervical Fluid Type: ________   Basal Body Temp: _______

Grooming Log

[ ] Shave   [ ] Wax   [ ] Thread   [ ] Laser

Intensity Scale: 1   2   3   4   5

Daily Habits & Triggers

Movement Goal: [ ] Done!

Mood: 1   2   3   4   5   Energy: 1   2   3   4   5

Caffeine: Alcohol:

The Evidence (150+ Connection)

Symptoms Noticed: ____

Food/Supplements: ____

Daily Vitality Log

The Morning Baseline

Date: _____/_____/________   Date of Cycle: _____/_____/________

Blood Pressure: _____ / _____

Waking Glucose: ___________   Weight: _____________

The PCOS Cycle Tracker

Flow: [ ] Light   [ ] Med   [ ] Heavy   [ ] Spotting

Ovulation Test: [ ] Positive   [ ] Negative

Cervical Fluid Type: _________   Basal Body Temp: ________

Grooming Log

[ ] Shave   [ ] Wax   [ ] Thread   [ ] Laser

Intensity Scale: 1   2   3   4   5

Daily Habits & Triggers

Movement Goal: [ ] Done!

Mood: 1   2   3   4   5   Energy: 1   2   3   4   5

Caffeine: Alcohol:

The Evidence (150+ Connection)

Symptoms Noticed: ____

Food/Supplements: ____

Daily Vitality Log

The Morning Baseline

Date: _____/______/_______   Date of Cycle: _____/______/________

Blood Pressure: ____ / ____

Waking Glucose: __________   Weight: ____________

The PCOS Cycle Tracker

Flow: [ ] Light   [ ] Med   [ ] Heavy   [ ] Spotting

Ovulation Test: [ ] Positive   [ ] Negative

Cervical Fluid Type: ________   Basal Body Temp: _______

Grooming Log

[ ] Shave   [ ] Wax   [ ] Thread   [ ] Laser

Intensity Scale: 1   2   3   4   5

Daily Habits & Triggers

Movement Goal: [ ] Done!

Mood: 1   2   3   4   5   Energy: 1   2   3   4   5

Caffeine: Alcohol:

The Evidence (150+ Connection)

Symptoms Noticed: ____

Food/Supplements: ____

Daily Vitality Log

The Morning Baseline

Date: _____/______/_______   Date of Cycle: _____/______/_______

Blood Pressure: _____ / _____

Waking Glucose: ___________   Weight: ____________

The PCOS Cycle Tracker

Flow: [ ] Light   [ ] Med   [ ] Heavy   [ ] Spotting

Ovulation Test: [ ] Positive   [ ] Negative

Cervical Fluid Type: _________   Basal Body Temp: ________

Grooming Log

[ ] Shave   [ ] Wax   [ ] Thread   [ ] Laser

Intensity Scale: 1   2   3   4   5

Daily Habits & Triggers

Movement Goal: [ ] Done!

Mood: 1   2   3   4   5   Energy: 1   2   3   4   5

Caffeine: Alcohol:

The Evidence (150+ Connection)

Symptoms Noticed: ____

Food/Supplements: ____

Daily Vitality Log

The Morning Baseline

Date: _____/______/________   Date of Cycle: _____/______/________

Blood Pressure: ____ / ____

Waking Glucose: __________   Weight: ____________

The PCOS Cycle Tracker

Flow: [ ] Light   [ ] Med   [ ] Heavy   [ ] Spotting

Ovulation Test: [ ] Positive   [ ] Negative

Cervical Fluid Type: _________   Basal Body Temp: ________

Grooming Log

[ ] Shave   [ ] Wax   [ ] Thread   [ ] Laser

Intensity Scale: 1   2   3   4   5

Daily Habits & Triggers

Movement Goal: [ ] Done!

Mood: 1   2   3   4   5   Energy: 1   2   3   4   5

Caffeine: Alcohol:

The Evidence (150+ Connection)

Symptoms Noticed: ____

Food/Supplements: ____

Daily Vitality Log

The Morning Baseline

Date: ______/______/________   Date of Cycle: ______/______/________

Blood Pressure: _____ / _____

Waking Glucose: ___________   Weight: ____________

The PCOS Cycle Tracker

Flow: [ ] Light   [ ] Med   [ ] Heavy   [ ] Spotting

Ovulation Test: [ ] Positive   [ ] Negative

Cervical Fluid Type: _________   Basal Body Temp: ________

Grooming Log

[ ] Shave   [ ] Wax   [ ] Thread   [ ] Laser

Intensity Scale: 1   2   3   4   5

Daily Habits & Triggers

Movement Goal: [ ] Done!

Mood: 1   2   3   4   5   Energy: 1   2   3   4   5

Caffeine: Alcohol:

The Evidence (150+ Connection)

Symptoms Noticed: ____

Food/Supplements: ____

Daily Vitality Log

The Morning Baseline

Date: _____/______/_______   Date of Cycle: ______/______/________

Blood Pressure: ____ / ____

Waking Glucose: __________   Weight: ___________

The PCOS Cycle Tracker

Flow: [] Light   [] Med   [] Heavy   [] Spotting

Ovulation Test: [] Positive   [] Negative

Cervical Fluid Type: _________   Basal Body Temp: ________

Grooming Log

[] Shave   [] Wax   [] Thread   [] Laser

Intensity Scale: 1   2   3   4   5

Daily Habits & Triggers

Movement Goal: [] Done!

Mood: 1   2   3   4   5   Energy: 1   2   3   4   5

Caffeine: Alcohol:

The Evidence (150+ Connection)

Symptoms Noticed: ____

Food/Supplements: ____

Daily Vitality Log

The Morning Baseline

Date: _____/_____/_______   Date of Cycle: _____/_____/________

Blood Pressure: _____ / _____

Waking Glucose: __________   Weight: ___________

The PCOS Cycle Tracker

Flow: [ ] Light   [ ] Med   [ ] Heavy   [ ] Spotting

Ovulation Test: [ ] Positive   [ ] Negative

Cervical Fluid Type: _________   Basal Body Temp: _______

Grooming Log

[ ] Shave   [ ] Wax   [ ] Thread   [ ] Laser

Intensity Scale: 1   2   3   4   5

Daily Habits & Triggers

Movement Goal: [ ] Done!

Mood: 1   2   3   4   5   Energy: 1   2   3   4   5

Caffeine: Alcohol:

The Evidence (150+ Connection)

Symptoms Noticed: ____

Food/Supplements: ____

Daily Vitality Log

The Morning Baseline

Date: _____/_____/_______   Date of Cycle: _____/_____/________

Blood Pressure: ____ / ____

Waking Glucose: __________   Weight: ___________

The PCOS Cycle Tracker

Flow: [] Light   [] Med   [] Heavy   [] Spotting

Ovulation Test: [] Positive   [] Negative

Cervical Fluid Type: _________   Basal Body Temp: ________

Grooming Log

[] Shave   [] Wax   [] Thread   [] Laser

Intensity Scale: 1   2   3   4   5

Daily Habits & Triggers

Movement Goal: [] Done!

Mood: 1   2   3   4   5   Energy: 1   2   3   4   5

Caffeine: Alcohol:

The Evidence (150+ Connection)

Symptoms Noticed: ____

Food/Supplements: ____

Daily Vitality Log

The Morning Baseline

Date: ______/______/________   Date of Cycle: ______/______/________

Blood Pressure: ____ / ____

Waking Glucose: __________   Weight: ___________

The PCOS Cycle Tracker

Flow: [ ] Light   [ ] Med   [ ] Heavy   [ ] Spotting

Ovulation Test: [ ] Positive   [ ] Negative

Cervical Fluid Type: _________   Basal Body Temp: ________

Grooming Log

[ ] Shave   [ ] Wax   [ ] Thread   [ ] Laser

Intensity Scale: 1   2   3   4   5

Daily Habits & Triggers

Movement Goal: [ ] Done!

Mood: 1   2   3   4   5   Energy: 1   2   3   4   5

Caffeine: Alcohol:

The Evidence (150+ Connection)

Symptoms Noticed: ____

Food/Supplements: ____

Daily Vitality Log

The Morning Baseline

Date: _____/______/________   Date of Cycle: _____/______/________

Blood Pressure: ____ / ____

Waking Glucose: ___________   Weight: ____________

The PCOS Cycle Tracker

Flow: [ ] Light   [ ] Med   [ ] Heavy   [ ] Spotting

Ovulation Test: [ ] Positive   [ ] Negative

Cervical Fluid Type: _________   Basal Body Temp: ________

Grooming Log

[ ] Shave   [ ] Wax   [ ] Thread   [ ] Laser

Intensity Scale: 1   2   3   4   5

Daily Habits & Triggers

Movement Goal: [ ] Done!

Mood: 1   2   3   4   5   Energy: 1   2   3   4   5

Caffeine: Alcohol:

The Evidence (150+ Connection)

Symptoms Noticed: ____

Food/Supplements: ____

Daily Vitality Log

The Morning Baseline

Date: _____/_____/_______   Date of Cycle: _____/_____/________

Blood Pressure: _____ / _____

Waking Glucose: __________   Weight: ____________

The PCOS Cycle Tracker

Flow: [ ] Light   [ ] Med   [ ] Heavy   [ ] Spotting

Ovulation Test: [ ] Positive   [ ] Negative

Cervical Fluid Type: _________   Basal Body Temp: ________

Grooming Log

[ ] Shave   [ ] Wax   [ ] Thread   [ ] Laser

Intensity Scale: 1   2   3   4   5

Daily Habits & Triggers

Movement Goal: [ ] Done!

Mood: 1   2   3   4   5   Energy: 1   2   3   4   5

Caffeine: Alcohol:

The Evidence (150+ Connection)

Symptoms Noticed: ____

Food/Supplements: ____

Daily Vitality Log

The Morning Baseline

Date: _____/_____/_______   Date of Cycle: _____/_____/_______

Blood Pressure: ____ / ____

Waking Glucose: __________   Weight: ____________

The PCOS Cycle Tracker

Flow: [] Light   [] Med   [] Heavy   [] Spotting

Ovulation Test: [] Positive   [] Negative

Cervical Fluid Type: _________   Basal Body Temp: _______

Grooming Log

[] Shave   [] Wax   [] Thread   [] Laser

Intensity Scale: 1   2   3   4   5

Daily Habits & Triggers

Movement Goal: [] Done!

Mood: 1   2   3   4   5   Energy: 1   2   3   4   5

Caffeine: Alcohol:

The Evidence (150+ Connection)

Symptoms Noticed: ____

Food/Supplements: ____

Daily Vitality Log

The Morning Baseline

Date: _____/_____/_______   Date of Cycle: _____/_____/_______

Blood Pressure: ____ / ____

Waking Glucose: __________   Weight: ____________

The PCOS Cycle Tracker

Flow: [ ] Light   [ ] Med   [ ] Heavy   [ ] Spotting

Ovulation Test: [ ] Positive   [ ] Negative

Cervical Fluid Type: _________   Basal Body Temp: ________

Grooming Log

[ ] Shave   [ ] Wax   [ ] Thread   [ ] Laser

Intensity Scale: 1   2   3   4   5

Daily Habits & Triggers

Movement Goal: [ ] Done!

Mood: 1   2   3   4   5   Energy: 1   2   3   4   5

Caffeine: Alcohol:

The Evidence (150+ Connection)

Symptoms Noticed: ____

Food/Supplements: ____

Daily Vitality Log

The Morning Baseline

Date: _____/_____/_______   Date of Cycle: _____/_____/_______

Blood Pressure: ____ / ____

Waking Glucose: __________   Weight: ____________

The PCOS Cycle Tracker

Flow: [ ] Light   [ ] Med   [ ] Heavy   [ ] Spotting

Ovulation Test: [ ] Positive   [ ] Negative

Cervical Fluid Type: _________   Basal Body Temp: _______

Grooming Log

[ ] Shave   [ ] Wax   [ ] Thread   [ ] Laser

Intensity Scale: 1   2   3   4   5

Daily Habits & Triggers

Movement Goal: [ ] Done!

Mood: 1   2   3   4   5   Energy: 1   2   3   4   5

Caffeine: Alcohol:

The Evidence (150+ Connection)

Symptoms Noticed: ____

Food/Supplements: ____

Daily Vitality Log

The Morning Baseline

Date: _____/_____/______   Date of Cycle: _____/_____/______

Blood Pressure: _____ / _____

Waking Glucose: __________   Weight: ___________

The PCOS Cycle Tracker

Flow: [ ] Light   [ ] Med   [ ] Heavy   [ ] Spotting

Ovulation Test: [ ] Positive   [ ] Negative

Cervical Fluid Type: _________   Basal Body Temp: _______

Grooming Log

[ ] Shave   [ ] Wax   [ ] Thread   [ ] Laser

Intensity Scale: 1   2   3   4   5

Daily Habits & Triggers

Movement Goal: [ ] Done!

Mood: 1   2   3   4   5   Energy: 1   2   3   4   5

Caffeine: Alcohol:

The Evidence (150+ Connection)

Symptoms Noticed: ____

Food/Supplements: ____

Daily Vitality Log

The Morning Baseline

Date: _____/______/_______   Date of Cycle: _____/______/________

Blood Pressure: _____ / _____

Waking Glucose: ___________   Weight: _____________

The PCOS Cycle Tracker

Flow: [ ] Light   [ ] Med   [ ] Heavy   [ ] Spotting

Ovulation Test: [ ] Positive   [ ] Negative

Cervical Fluid Type: _________   Basal Body Temp: ________

Grooming Log

[ ] Shave   [ ] Wax   [ ] Thread   [ ] Laser

Intensity Scale: 1   2   3   4   5

Daily Habits & Triggers

Movement Goal: [ ] Done!

Mood: 1   2   3   4   5   Energy: 1   2   3   4   5

Caffeine: Alcohol:

The Evidence (150+ Connection)

Symptoms Noticed: ____

Food/Supplements: ____

Daily Vitality Log

The Morning Baseline

Date: _____/______/________   Date of Cycle: ______/______/_________

Blood Pressure: _____ / _____

Waking Glucose: ___________   Weight: _____________

The PCOS Cycle Tracker

Flow: [ ] Light   [ ] Med   [ ] Heavy   [ ] Spotting

Ovulation Test: [ ] Positive   [ ] Negative

Cervical Fluid Type: _________   Basal Body Temp: ________

Grooming Log

[ ] Shave   [ ] Wax   [ ] Thread   [ ] Laser

Intensity Scale: 1   2   3   4   5

Daily Habits & Triggers

Movement Goal: [ ] Done!

Mood: 1   2   3   4   5   Energy: 1   2   3   4   5

Caffeine: Alcohol:

The Evidence (150+ Connection)

Symptoms Noticed: ____

Food/Supplements: ____

Daily Vitality Log

The Morning Baseline

Date: _____/______/________   Date of Cycle: _____/______/________

Blood Pressure: ____ / ____

Waking Glucose: __________   Weight: ____________

The PCOS Cycle Tracker

Flow: [] Light   [] Med   [] Heavy   [] Spotting

Ovulation Test: [] Positive   [] Negative

Cervical Fluid Type: _________   Basal Body Temp: ________

Grooming Log

[] Shave   [] Wax   [] Thread   [] Laser

Intensity Scale: 1   2   3   4   5

Daily Habits & Triggers

Movement Goal: [] Done!

Mood: 1   2   3   4   5   Energy: 1   2   3   4   5

Caffeine: Alcohol:

The Evidence (150+ Connection)

Symptoms Noticed: ____

Food/Supplements: ____

Daily Vitality Log

The Morning Baseline

Date: _____/_____/_________   Date of Cycle: _____/_____/_________

♥ Blood Pressure: _____ / _____

Waking Glucose: ___________   Weight: ___________

The PCOS Cycle Tracker

Flow: [ ] Light   [ ] Med   [ ] Heavy   [ ] Spotting

Ovulation Test: [ ] Positive   [ ] Negative

Cervical Fluid Type: _________   Basal Body Temp: _________

Grooming Log

[ ] Shave   [ ] Wax   [ ] Thread   [ ] Laser

Intensity Scale: 1   2   3   4   5

Daily Habits & Triggers

Movement Goal: [ ] Done!

Mood: 1   2   3   4   5   Energy: 1   2   3   4   5

Caffeine: Alcohol:

The Evidence (150+ Connection)

Symptoms Noticed: ____

Food/Supplements: ____

Daily Vitality Log

The Morning Baseline

Date: _____/_____/_______   Date of Cycle: _____/_____/________

Blood Pressure: ____ / ____

Waking Glucose: __________   Weight: ____________

The PCOS Cycle Tracker

Flow: [ ] Light   [ ] Med   [ ] Heavy   [ ] Spotting

Ovulation Test: [ ] Positive   [ ] Negative

Cervical Fluid Type: _________   Basal Body Temp: ________

Grooming Log

[ ] Shave   [ ] Wax   [ ] Thread   [ ] Laser

Intensity Scale: 1   2   3   4   5

Daily Habits & Triggers

Movement Goal: [ ] Done!

Mood: 1   2   3   4   5   Energy: 1   2   3   4   5

Caffeine: Alcohol:

The Evidence (150+ Connection)

Symptoms Noticed: ____

Food/Supplements: ____

Daily Vitality Log

The Morning Baseline

Date: _____/_____/_______   Date of Cycle: _____/_____/_______

Blood Pressure: _____/ _____

Waking Glucose: __________   Weight: ____________

The PCOS Cycle Tracker

Flow: [] Light   [] Med   [] Heavy   [] Spotting

Ovulation Test: [] Positive   [] Negative

Cervical Fluid Type: _________   Basal Body Temp: ________

Grooming Log

[] Shave   [] Wax   [] Thread   [] Laser

Intensity Scale: 1   2   3   4   5

Daily Habits & Triggers

Movement Goal: [] Done!

Mood: 1 2 3 4 5   Energy: 1 2 3 4 5

Caffeine: Alcohol:

The Evidence (150+ Connection)

Symptoms Noticed: ____

Food/Supplements: ____

Daily Vitality Log

The Morning Baseline

Date: _____/_____/______   Date of Cycle: _____/_____/______

Blood Pressure: ____ / ____

Waking Glucose: __________   Weight: __________

The PCOS Cycle Tracker

Flow: [ ] Light   [ ] Med   [ ] Heavy   [ ] Spotting

Ovulation Test: [ ] Positive   [ ] Negative

Cervical Fluid Type: ________   Basal Body Temp: _______

Grooming Log

[ ] Shave   [ ] Wax   [ ] Thread   [ ] Laser

Intensity Scale: 1   2   3   4   5

Daily Habits & Triggers

Movement Goal: [ ] Done!

Mood: 1   2   3   4   5   Energy: 1   2   3   4   5

Caffeine: Alcohol:

The Evidence (150+ Connection)

Symptoms Noticed: ____

Food/Supplements: ____

Daily Vitality Log

The Morning Baseline

Date: _____/_____/_______   Date of Cycle: _____/_____/________

Blood Pressure: ____ / ____

Waking Glucose: __________   Weight: ____________

The PCOS Cycle Tracker

Flow: [ ] Light   [ ] Med   [ ] Heavy   [ ] Spotting

Ovulation Test: [ ] Positive   [ ] Negative

Cervical Fluid Type: _________   Basal Body Temp: ________

Grooming Log

[ ] Shave   [ ] Wax   [ ] Thread   [ ] Laser

Intensity Scale: 1   2   3   4   5

Daily Habits & Triggers

Movement Goal: [ ] Done!

Mood: 1   2   3   4   5   Energy: 1   2   3   4   5

Caffeine: Alcohol:

The Evidence (150+ Connection)

Symptoms Noticed: ____

Food/Supplements: ____

Daily Vitality Log

The Morning Baseline

Date: _____/_____/________   Date of Cycle: _____/_____/________

Blood Pressure: _____ / _____

Waking Glucose: __________   Weight: ___________

The PCOS Cycle Tracker

Flow: [] Light   [] Med   [] Heavy   [] Spotting

Ovulation Test: [] Positive   [] Negative

Cervical Fluid Type: _________   Basal Body Temp: _______

Grooming Log

[] Shave   [] Wax   [] Thread   [] Laser

Intensity Scale: 1   2   3   4   5

Daily Habits & Triggers

Movement Goal: [] Done!

Mood: 1   2   3   4   5   Energy: 1   2   3   4   5

Caffeine: Alcohol:

The Evidence (150+ Connection)

Symptoms Noticed: ____

Food/Supplements: ____

Daily Vitality Log

The Morning Baseline

Date: _____/_____/______   Date of Cycle: _____/_____/________

❤️ Blood Pressure: _____ / _____

Waking Glucose: __________   Weight: ___________

The PCOS Cycle Tracker

Flow: [ ] Light   [ ] Med   [ ] Heavy   [ ] Spotting

Ovulation Test: [ ] Positive   [ ] Negative

Cervical Fluid Type: _________   Basal Body Temp: ________

Grooming Log

[ ] Shave   [ ] Wax   [ ] Thread   [ ] Laser

Intensity Scale: 1   2   3   4   5

Daily Habits & Triggers

Movement Goal: [ ] Done!

Mood: 1   2   3   4   5   Energy: 1   2   3   4   5

Caffeine: Alcohol:

The Evidence (150+ Connection)

Symptoms Noticed: ____

Food/Supplements: ____

Daily Vitality Log

The Morning Baseline

Date: _____/_____/_______   Date of Cycle: _____/_____/________

Blood Pressure: ____ / ____

Waking Glucose: __________   Weight: ___________

The PCOS Cycle Tracker

Flow: [ ] Light   [ ] Med   [ ] Heavy   [ ] Spotting

Ovulation Test: [ ] Positive   [ ] Negative

Cervical Fluid Type: _________   Basal Body Temp: _______

Grooming Log

[ ] Shave   [ ] Wax   [ ] Thread   [ ] Laser

Intensity Scale: 1   2   3   4   5

Daily Habits & Triggers

Movement Goal: [ ] Done!

Mood: 1   2   3   4   5   Energy: 1   2   3   4   5

Caffeine: Alcohol:

The Evidence (150+ Connection)

Symptoms Noticed: ____

Food/Supplements: ____

Daily Vitality Log

The Morning Baseline

Date: _____/______/_______   Date of Cycle: _____/______/________

Blood Pressure: _____ / _____

Waking Glucose: ___________   Weight: ____________

The PCOS Cycle Tracker

Flow: [ ] Light   [ ] Med   [ ] Heavy   [ ] Spotting

Ovulation Test: [ ] Positive   [ ] Negative

Cervical Fluid Type: _________   Basal Body Temp: ________

Grooming Log

[ ] Shave   [ ] Wax   [ ] Thread   [ ] Laser

Intensity Scale: 1   2   3   4   5

Daily Habits & Triggers

Movement Goal: [ ] Done!

Mood: 1   2   3   4   5   Energy: 1   2   3   4   5

Caffeine: Alcohol:

The Evidence (150+ Connection)

Symptoms Noticed: ____

Food/Supplements: ____

Daily Vitality Log

The Morning Baseline

Date: _____/______/________   Date of Cycle: _____/______/________

Blood Pressure: _____ / _____

Waking Glucose: ___________   Weight: ____________

The PCOS Cycle Tracker

Flow: [ ] Light   [ ] Med   [ ] Heavy   [ ] Spotting

Ovulation Test: [ ] Positive   [ ] Negative

Cervical Fluid Type: _________   Basal Body Temp: ________

Grooming Log

[ ] Shave   [ ] Wax   [ ] Thread   [ ] Laser

Intensity Scale: 1   2   3   4   5

Daily Habits & Triggers

Movement Goal: [ ] Done!

Mood: 1   2   3   4   5   Energy: 1   2   3   4   5

Caffeine: Alcohol:

The Evidence (150+ Connection)

Symptoms Noticed: ____

Food/Supplements: ____

Daily Vitality Log

The Morning Baseline

Date: _____/_____/_______   Date of Cycle: _____/_____/________

Blood Pressure: _____ / _____

Waking Glucose: __________   Weight: ___________

The PCOS Cycle Tracker

Flow: [ ] Light   [ ] Med   [ ] Heavy   [ ] Spotting

Ovulation Test: [ ] Positive   [ ] Negative

Cervical Fluid Type: _________   Basal Body Temp: ________

Grooming Log

[ ] Shave   [ ] Wax   [ ] Thread   [ ] Laser

Intensity Scale: 1   2   3   4   5

Daily Habits & Triggers

Movement Goal: [ ] Done!

Mood: 1   2   3   4   5   Energy: 1   2   3   4   5

Caffeine: Alcohol:

The Evidence (150+ Connection)

Symptoms Noticed: ____

Food/Supplements: ____

Daily Vitality Log

The Morning Baseline

Date: _______/_______/_________   Date of Cycle: _______/_______/_________

Blood Pressure: ______ / ______

Waking Glucose: ___________   Weight: _____________

The PCOS Cycle Tracker

Flow: [ ] Light   [ ] Med   [ ] Heavy   [ ] Spotting

Ovulation Test: [ ] Positive   [ ] Negative

Cervical Fluid Type: __________   Basal Body Temp: _________

Grooming Log

[ ] Shave   [ ] Wax   [ ] Thread   [ ] Laser

Intensity Scale: 1   2   3   4   5

Daily Habits & Triggers

Movement Goal: [ ] Done!

Mood: 1   2   3   4   5   Energy: 1   2   3   4   5

Caffeine: Alcohol:

The Evidence (150+ Connection)

Symptoms Noticed: ____

Food/Supplements: ____

Daily Vitality Log

The Morning Baseline

Date: _____/_____/_______   Date of Cycle: _____/_____/_______

Blood Pressure: _____ / _____

Waking Glucose: __________   Weight: ___________

The PCOS Cycle Tracker

Flow: [ ] Light   [ ] Med   [ ] Heavy   [ ] Spotting

Ovulation Test: [ ] Positive   [ ] Negative

Cervical Fluid Type: _________   Basal Body Temp: ________

Grooming Log

[ ] Shave   [ ] Wax   [ ] Thread   [ ] Laser

Intensity Scale: 1   2   3   4   5

Daily Habits & Triggers

Movement Goal: [ ] Done!

Mood: 1   2   3   4   5   Energy: 1   2   3   4   5

Caffeine: Alcohol:

The Evidence (150+ Connection)

Symptoms Noticed: ____

Food/Supplements: ____

Daily Vitality Log

The Morning Baseline

Date: _____/_____/_______   Date of Cycle: _____/_____/________

Blood Pressure: ____ / ____

Waking Glucose: __________   Weight: ____________

The PCOS Cycle Tracker

Flow: [ ] Light   [ ] Med   [ ] Heavy   [ ] Spotting

Ovulation Test: [ ] Positive   [ ] Negative

Cervical Fluid Type: _________   Basal Body Temp: ________

Grooming Log

[ ] Shave   [ ] Wax   [ ] Thread   [ ] Laser

Intensity Scale: 1   2   3   4   5

Daily Habits & Triggers

Movement Goal: [ ] Done!

Mood: 1   2   3   4   5   Energy: 1   2   3   4   5

Caffeine: Alcohol:

The Evidence (150+ Connection)

Symptoms Noticed: ____

Food/Supplements: ____

Daily Vitality Log

The Morning Baseline

Date: _____/______/_______   Date of Cycle: _____/______/________

Blood Pressure: ____/____

Waking Glucose: __________   Weight: ____________

The PCOS Cycle Tracker

Flow: [ ] Light   [ ] Med   [ ] Heavy   [ ] Spotting

Ovulation Test: [ ] Positive   [ ] Negative

Cervical Fluid Type: _________   Basal Body Temp: ________

Grooming Log

[ ] Shave   [ ] Wax   [ ] Thread   [ ] Laser

Intensity Scale: 1   2   3   4   5

Daily Habits & Triggers

Movement Goal: [ ] Done!

Mood: 1   2   3   4   5   Energy: 1   2   3   4   5

Caffeine: Alcohol:

The Evidence (150+ Connection)

Symptoms Noticed: ____

Food/Supplements: ____

Daily Vitality Log

The Morning Baseline

Date: _____/_______/________   Date of Cycle: ______/_______/_________

Blood Pressure: _____ / _____

Waking Glucose: ___________   Weight: ____________

The PCOS Cycle Tracker

Flow: [ ] Light   [ ] Med   [ ] Heavy   [ ] Spotting

Ovulation Test: [ ] Positive   [ ] Negative

Cervical Fluid Type: _________   Basal Body Temp: ________

Grooming Log

[ ] Shave   [ ] Wax   [ ] Thread   [ ] Laser

Intensity Scale: 1   2   3   4   5

Daily Habits & Triggers

Movement Goal: [ ] Done!

Mood: 1   2   3   4   5   Energy: 1   2   3   4   5

Caffeine: Alcohol:

The Evidence (150+ Connection)

Symptoms Noticed: ____

Food/Supplements: ____

Daily Vitality Log

The Morning Baseline

Date: _____/_____/_______   Date of Cycle: _____/_____/________

Blood Pressure: _____ / _____

Waking Glucose: __________   Weight: ___________

The PCOS Cycle Tracker

Flow: [ ] Light   [ ] Med   [ ] Heavy   [ ] Spotting

Ovulation Test: [ ] Positive   [ ] Negative

Cervical Fluid Type: _________   Basal Body Temp: ________

Grooming Log

[ ] Shave   [ ] Wax   [ ] Thread   [ ] Laser

Intensity Scale: 1   2   3   4   5

Daily Habits & Triggers

Movement Goal: [ ] Done!

Mood: 1   2   3   4   5   Energy: 1   2   3   4   5

Caffeine: Alcohol:

The Evidence (150+ Connection)

Symptoms Noticed: ____

Food/Supplements: ____

Daily Vitality Log

The Morning Baseline

Date: _____/_____/______   Date of Cycle: _____/_____/_______

Blood Pressure: ____ / ____

Waking Glucose: __________   Weight: ___________

The PCOS Cycle Tracker

Flow: [ ] Light   [ ] Med   [ ] Heavy   [ ] Spotting

Ovulation Test: [ ] Positive   [ ] Negative

Cervical Fluid Type: _________   Basal Body Temp: _______

Grooming Log

[ ] Shave   [ ] Wax   [ ] Thread   [ ] Laser

Intensity Scale: 1   2   3   4   5

Daily Habits & Triggers

Movement Goal: [ ] Done!

Mood: 1   2   3   4   5   Energy: 1   2   3   4   5

Caffeine: Alcohol:

The Evidence (150+ Connection)

Symptoms Noticed: ____

Food/Supplements: ____

Daily Vitality Log

The Morning Baseline

Date: _____/_____/_______   Date of Cycle: _____/_____/_______

Blood Pressure: _____/_____

Waking Glucose: __________   Weight: __________

The PCOS Cycle Tracker

Flow: [ ] Light   [ ] Med   [ ] Heavy   [ ] Spotting

Ovulation Test: [ ] Positive   [ ] Negative

Cervical Fluid Type: ________   Basal Body Temp: ________

Grooming Log

[ ] Shave   [ ] Wax   [ ] Thread   [ ] Laser

Intensity Scale: 1   2   3   4   5

Daily Habits & Triggers

Movement Goal: [ ] Done!

Mood: 1   2   3   4   5   Energy: 1   2   3   4   5

Caffeine: Alcohol:

The Evidence (150+ Connection)

Symptoms Noticed: ____

Food/Supplements: ____

Daily Vitality Log

The Morning Baseline

Date: _____ / _____ / _______   Date of Cycle: _____ / _____ / _______

Blood Pressure: _____ / _____

Waking Glucose: __________   Weight: ___________

The PCOS Cycle Tracker

Flow: [ ] Light   [ ] Med   [ ] Heavy   [ ] Spotting

Ovulation Test: [ ] Positive   [ ] Negative

Cervical Fluid Type: _________   Basal Body Temp: _______

Grooming Log

[ ] Shave   [ ] Wax   [ ] Thread   [ ] Laser

Intensity Scale: 1   2   3   4   5

Daily Habits & Triggers

Movement Goal: [ ] Done!

Mood: 1   2   3   4   5   Energy: 1   2   3   4   5

Caffeine: Alcohol:

The Evidence (150+ Connection)

Symptoms Noticed: ____

Food/Supplements: ____

Daily Vitality Log

The Morning Baseline

Date: _____/______/_______   Date of Cycle: ______/______/________

Blood Pressure: _____ / ____

Waking Glucose: __________   Weight: ____________

The PCOS Cycle Tracker

Flow: [ ] Light   [ ] Med   [ ] Heavy   [ ] Spotting

Ovulation Test: [ ] Positive   [ ] Negative

Cervical Fluid Type: _________   Basal Body Temp: ________

Grooming Log

[ ] Shave   [ ] Wax   [ ] Thread   [ ] Laser

Intensity Scale: 1   2   3   4   5

Daily Habits & Triggers

Movement Goal: [ ] Done!

Mood: 1   2   3   4   5   Energy: 1   2   3   4   5

Caffeine: Alcohol:

The Evidence (150+ Connection)

Symptoms Noticed: ____

Food/Supplements: ____

Daily Vitality Log

The Morning Baseline

Date: _____/______/_______   Date of Cycle: _____/______/________

Blood Pressure: ____ / ____

Waking Glucose: __________   Weight: ___________

The PCOS Cycle Tracker

Flow: [ ] Light   [ ] Med   [ ] Heavy   [ ] Spotting

Ovulation Test: [ ] Positive   [ ] Negative

Cervical Fluid Type: _________   Basal Body Temp: ________

Grooming Log

[ ] Shave   [ ] Wax   [ ] Thread   [ ] Laser

Intensity Scale: 1   2   3   4   5

Daily Habits & Triggers

Movement Goal: [ ] Done!

Mood: 1   2   3   4   5   Energy: 1   2   3   4   5

Caffeine: Alcohol:

The Evidence (150+ Connection)

Symptoms Noticed: ____

Food/Supplements: ____

Daily Vitality Log

The Morning Baseline

Date: _____/______/_______   Date of Cycle: ______/______/________

Blood Pressure: _____ / _____

Waking Glucose: ___________   Weight: _____________

The PCOS Cycle Tracker

Flow: [ ] Light   [ ] Med   [ ] Heavy   [ ] Spotting

Ovulation Test: [ ] Positive   [ ] Negative

Cervical Fluid Type: _________   Basal Body Temp: ________

Grooming Log

[ ] Shave   [ ] Wax   [ ] Thread   [ ] Laser

Intensity Scale: 1   2   3   4   5

Daily Habits & Triggers

Movement Goal: [ ] Done!

Mood: 1   2   3   4   5   Energy: 1   2   3   4   5

Caffeine: Alcohol:

The Evidence (150+ Connection)

Symptoms Noticed: ____

Food/Supplements: ____

Daily Vitality Log

The Morning Baseline

Date: _____/_____/_______   Date of Cycle: _____/_____/_______

Blood Pressure: ____ / ____

Waking Glucose: __________   Weight: ___________

The PCOS Cycle Tracker

Flow: [ ] Light   [ ] Med   [ ] Heavy   [ ] Spotting

Ovulation Test: [ ] Positive   [ ] Negative

Cervical Fluid Type: _________   Basal Body Temp: _______

Grooming Log

[ ] Shave   [ ] Wax   [ ] Thread   [ ] Laser

Intensity Scale: 1   2   3   4   5

Daily Habits & Triggers

Movement Goal: [ ] Done!

Mood: 1   2   3   4   5   Energy: 1   2   3   4   5

Caffeine: Alcohol:

The Evidence (150+ Connection)

Symptoms Noticed: ____

Food/Supplements: ____

Daily Vitality Log

The Morning Baseline

Date: _____/_____/_______   Date of Cycle: _____/_____/________

Blood Pressure: _____ / _____

Waking Glucose: ___________   Weight: ____________

The PCOS Cycle Tracker

Flow: [ ] Light   [ ] Med   [ ] Heavy   [ ] Spotting

Ovulation Test: [ ] Positive   [ ] Negative

Cervical Fluid Type: __________   Basal Body Temp: ________

Grooming Log

[ ] Shave   [ ] Wax   [ ] Thread   [ ] Laser

Intensity Scale: 1   2   3   4   5

Daily Habits & Triggers

Movement Goal: [ ] Done!

Mood: 1   2   3   4   5   Energy: 1   2   3   4   5

Caffeine: Alcohol:

The Evidence (150+ Connection)

Symptoms Noticed: ____

Food/Supplements: ____

Daily Vitality Log

The Morning Baseline

Date: _____/_____/_______   Date of Cycle: _____/_____/_______

Blood Pressure: _____ / _____

Waking Glucose: __________   Weight: ___________

The PCOS Cycle Tracker

Flow: [ ] Light   [ ] Med   [ ] Heavy   [ ] Spotting

Ovulation Test: [ ] Positive   [ ] Negative

Cervical Fluid Type: _________   Basal Body Temp: _______

Grooming Log

[ ] Shave   [ ] Wax   [ ] Thread   [ ] Laser

Intensity Scale: 1   2   3   4   5

Daily Habits & Triggers

Movement Goal: [ ] Done!

Mood: 1   2   3   4   5   Energy: 1   2   3   4   5

Caffeine: Alcohol:

The Evidence (150+ Connection)

Symptoms Noticed: ____

Food/Supplements: ____

Daily Vitality Log

The Morning Baseline

Date: _____/_____/_______   Date of Cycle: _____/_____/________

Blood Pressure: _____ / _____

Waking Glucose: ___________   Weight: ___________

The PCOS Cycle Tracker

Flow: [ ] Light   [ ] Med   [ ] Heavy   [ ] Spotting

Ovulation Test: [ ] Positive   [ ] Negative

Cervical Fluid Type: _________   Basal Body Temp: ________

Grooming Log

[ ] Shave   [ ] Wax   [ ] Thread   [ ] Laser

Intensity Scale: 1   2   3   4   5

Daily Habits & Triggers

Movement Goal: [ ] Done!

Mood: 1   2   3   4   5   Energy: 1   2   3   4   5

Caffeine: Alcohol:

The Evidence (150+ Connection)

Symptoms Noticed: ____

Food/Supplements: ____

Daily Vitality Log

The Morning Baseline

Date: _____/______/_______   Date of Cycle: _____/______/________

Blood Pressure: ____ / ____

Waking Glucose: __________   Weight: ____________

The PCOS Cycle Tracker

Flow: [ ] Light   [ ] Med   [ ] Heavy   [ ] Spotting

Ovulation Test: [ ] Positive   [ ] Negative

Cervical Fluid Type: _________   Basal Body Temp: ________

Grooming Log

[ ] Shave   [ ] Wax   [ ] Thread   [ ] Laser

Intensity Scale: 1   2   3   4   5

Daily Habits & Triggers

Movement Goal: [ ] Done!

Mood: 1   2   3   4   5   Energy: 1   2   3   4   5

Caffeine: Alcohol:

The Evidence (150+ Connection)

Symptoms Noticed: ____

Food/Supplements: ____

Daily Vitality Log

The Morning Baseline

Date: _____/_____/_______   Date of Cycle: _____/_____/________

Blood Pressure: _____ / _____

Waking Glucose: ___________   Weight: ____________

The PCOS Cycle Tracker

Flow: [ ] Light   [ ] Med   [ ] Heavy   [ ] Spotting

Ovulation Test: [ ] Positive   [ ] Negative

Cervical Fluid Type: __________   Basal Body Temp: ________

Grooming Log

[ ] Shave   [ ] Wax   [ ] Thread   [ ] Laser

Intensity Scale: 1   2   3   4   5

Daily Habits & Triggers

Movement Goal: [ ] Done!

Mood: 1   2   3   4   5   Energy: 1   2   3   4   5

Caffeine: Alcohol:

The Evidence (150+ Connection)

Symptoms Noticed: ____

Food/Supplements: ____

Daily Vitality Log

The Morning Baseline

Date: _____/______/_______   Date of Cycle: _____/______/________

Blood Pressure: ____ / ____

Waking Glucose: __________   Weight: ___________

The PCOS Cycle Tracker

Flow: [ ] Light   [ ] Med   [ ] Heavy   [ ] Spotting

Ovulation Test: [ ] Positive   [ ] Negative

Cervical Fluid Type: _________   Basal Body Temp: _______

Grooming Log

[ ] Shave   [ ] Wax   [ ] Thread   [ ] Laser

Intensity Scale: 1   2   3   4   5

Daily Habits & Triggers

Movement Goal: [ ] Done!

Mood: 1   2   3   4   5   Energy: 1   2   3   4   5

Caffeine: Alcohol:

The Evidence (150+ Connection)

Symptoms Noticed: ____

Food/Supplements: ____

Daily Vitality Log

The Morning Baseline

Date: _____/_____/_______   Date of Cycle: _____/_____/_______

Blood Pressure: _____ / _____

Waking Glucose: ___________   Weight: ___________

The PCOS Cycle Tracker

Flow: [ ] Light   [ ] Med   [ ] Heavy   [ ] Spotting

Ovulation Test: [ ] Positive   [ ] Negative

Cervical Fluid Type: _________   Basal Body Temp: _______

Grooming Log

[ ] Shave   [ ] Wax   [ ] Thread   [ ] Laser

Intensity Scale: 1   2   3   4   5

Daily Habits & Triggers

Movement Goal: [ ] Done!

Mood: 1   2   3   4   5   Energy: 1   2   3   4   5

Caffeine: Alcohol:

The Evidence (150+ Connection)

Symptoms Noticed: _______________________________________

Food/Supplements: _______________________________________

Daily Vitality Log

The Morning Baseline

Date: _____/_____/_______   Date of Cycle: _____/_____/________

Blood Pressure: _____ / _____

Waking Glucose: __________   Weight: ____________

The PCOS Cycle Tracker

Flow: [ ] Light   [ ] Med   [ ] Heavy   [ ] Spotting

Ovulation Test: [ ] Positive   [ ] Negative

Cervical Fluid Type: _________   Basal Body Temp: ________

Grooming Log

[ ] Shave   [ ] Wax   [ ] Thread   [ ] Laser

Intensity Scale: 1   2   3   4   5

Daily Habits & Triggers

Movement Goal: [ ] Done!

Mood: 1   2   3   4   5   Energy: 1   2   3   4   5

Caffeine: Alcohol:

The Evidence (150+ Connection)

Symptoms Noticed: ____

Food/Supplements: ____

Daily Vitality Log

The Morning Baseline

Date: _____/_____/_______   Date of Cycle: _____/_____/_______

Blood Pressure: _____ / _____

Waking Glucose: __________   Weight: ___________

The PCOS Cycle Tracker

Flow: [ ] Light   [ ] Med   [ ] Heavy   [ ] Spotting

Ovulation Test: [ ] Positive   [ ] Negative

Cervical Fluid Type: _________   Basal Body Temp: ________

Grooming Log

[ ] Shave   [ ] Wax   [ ] Thread   [ ] Laser

Intensity Scale: 1   2   3   4   5

Daily Habits & Triggers

Movement Goal: [ ] Done!

Mood: 1   2   3   4   5   Energy: 1   2   3   4   5

Caffeine: Alcohol:

The Evidence (150+ Connection)

Symptoms Noticed: ____

Food/Supplements: ____

Daily Vitality Log

The Morning Baseline

Date: _____/_____/_______   Date of Cycle: _____/_____/________

Blood Pressure: ____ / ____

Waking Glucose: __________   Weight: ___________

The PCOS Cycle Tracker

Flow: [ ] Light   [ ] Med   [ ] Heavy   [ ] Spotting

Ovulation Test: [ ] Positive   [ ] Negative

Cervical Fluid Type: ________   Basal Body Temp: _______

Grooming Log

[ ] Shave   [ ] Wax   [ ] Thread   [ ] Laser

Intensity Scale: 1   2   3   4   5

Daily Habits & Triggers

Movement Goal: [ ] Done!

Mood: 1   2   3   4   5   Energy: 1   2   3   4   5

Caffeine: Alcohol:

The Evidence (150+ Connection)

Symptoms Noticed: ____

Food/Supplements: ____

Daily Vitality Log

The Morning Baseline

Date: _____/______/________   Date of Cycle: ______/______/________

Blood Pressure: _____ / _____

Waking Glucose: ___________   Weight: _____________

The PCOS Cycle Tracker

Flow: [ ] Light   [ ] Med   [ ] Heavy   [ ] Spotting

Ovulation Test: [ ] Positive   [ ] Negative

Cervical Fluid Type: _________   Basal Body Temp: ________

Grooming Log

[ ] Shave   [ ] Wax   [ ] Thread   [ ] Laser

Intensity Scale: 1   2   3   4   5

Daily Habits & Triggers

Movement Goal: [ ] Done!

Mood: 1   2   3   4   5   Energy: 1   2   3   4   5

Caffeine: Alcohol:

The Evidence (150+ Connection)

Symptoms Noticed: ____

Food/Supplements: ____

Daily Vitality Log

The Morning Baseline

Date: _____/______/_______   Date of Cycle: _____/______/________

Blood Pressure: _____ / _____

Waking Glucose: __________   Weight: ____________

The PCOS Cycle Tracker

Flow: [ ] Light   [ ] Med   [ ] Heavy   [ ] Spotting

Ovulation Test: [ ] Positive   [ ] Negative

Cervical Fluid Type: _________   Basal Body Temp: _______

Grooming Log

[ ] Shave   [ ] Wax   [ ] Thread   [ ] Laser

Intensity Scale: 1   2   3   4   5

Daily Habits & Triggers

Movement Goal: [ ] Done!

Mood: 1   2   3   4   5   Energy: 1   2   3   4   5

Caffeine: Alcohol:

The Evidence (150+ Connection)

Symptoms Noticed: ____

Food/Supplements: ____

Daily Vitality Log

The Morning Baseline

Date: _____/_____/________   Date of Cycle: _____/_____/________

Blood Pressure: _____ / _____

Waking Glucose: __________   Weight: ____________

The PCOS Cycle Tracker

Flow: [ ] Light   [ ] Med   [ ] Heavy   [ ] Spotting

Ovulation Test: [ ] Positive   [ ] Negative

Cervical Fluid Type: __________   Basal Body Temp: ________

Grooming Log

[ ] Shave   [ ] Wax   [ ] Thread   [ ] Laser

Intensity Scale: 1   2   3   4   5

Daily Habits & Triggers

Movement Goal: [ ] Done!

Mood: 1   2   3   4   5   Energy: 1   2   3   4   5

Caffeine: Alcohol:

The Evidence (150+ Connection)

Symptoms Noticed: ____

Food/Supplements: ____

Daily Vitality Log

The Morning Baseline

Date: _____ /_____ /________   Date of Cycle: _____ /_____ /________

Blood Pressure: ____ / ____

Waking Glucose: __________   Weight: ___________

The PCOS Cycle Tracker

Flow: [ ] Light   [ ] Med   [ ] Heavy   [ ] Spotting

Ovulation Test: [ ] Positive   [ ] Negative

Cervical Fluid Type: _________   Basal Body Temp: ________

Grooming Log

[ ] Shave   [ ] Wax   [ ] Thread   [ ] Laser

Intensity Scale: 1   2   3   4   5

Daily Habits & Triggers

Movement Goal: [ ] Done!

Mood: 1   2   3   4   5   Energy: 1   2   3   4   5

Caffeine: Alcohol:

The Evidence (150+ Connection)

Symptoms Noticed: ____

Food/Supplements: ____

Daily Vitality Log

The Morning Baseline

Date: _____/______/_______   Date of Cycle: _____/______/_______

Blood Pressure: _____ / _____

Waking Glucose: ___________   Weight: _____________

The PCOS Cycle Tracker

Flow: [ ] Light   [ ] Med   [ ] Heavy   [ ] Spotting

Ovulation Test: [ ] Positive   [ ] Negative

Cervical Fluid Type: _________   Basal Body Temp: ________

Grooming Log

[ ] Shave   [ ] Wax   [ ] Thread   [ ] Laser

Intensity Scale: 1   2   3   4   5

Daily Habits & Triggers

Movement Goal: [ ] Done!

Mood: 1   2   3   4   5   Energy: 1   2   3   4   5

Caffeine: Alcohol:

The Evidence (150+ Connection)

Symptoms Noticed: ____

Food/Supplements: ____

Daily Vitality Log

The Morning Baseline

Date: _____/______/_______   Date of Cycle: _____/______/________

Blood Pressure: ____ / ____

Waking Glucose: __________   Weight: ___________

The PCOS Cycle Tracker

Flow: [ ] Light   [ ] Med   [ ] Heavy   [ ] Spotting

Ovulation Test: [ ] Positive   [ ] Negative

Cervical Fluid Type: _________   Basal Body Temp: ________

Grooming Log

[ ] Shave   [ ] Wax   [ ] Thread   [ ] Laser

Intensity Scale: 1   2   3   4   5

Daily Habits & Triggers

Movement Goal: [ ] Done!

Mood: 1   2   3   4   5   Energy: 1   2   3   4   5

Caffeine: Alcohol:

The Evidence (150+ Connection)

Symptoms Noticed: ____

Food/Supplements: ____

Daily Vitality Log

The Morning Baseline

Date: _____/_____/_______   Date of Cycle: _____/_____/_______

Blood Pressure: _____ / _____

Waking Glucose: ___________   Weight: ____________

The PCOS Cycle Tracker

Flow: [ ] Light   [ ] Med   [ ] Heavy   [ ] Spotting

Ovulation Test: [ ] Positive   [ ] Negative

Cervical Fluid Type: _________   Basal Body Temp: _______

Grooming Log

[ ] Shave   [ ] Wax   [ ] Thread   [ ] Laser

Intensity Scale: 1   2   3   4   5

Daily Habits & Triggers

Movement Goal: [ ] Done!

Mood: 1   2   3   4   5   Energy: 1   2   3   4   5

Caffeine: Alcohol:

The Evidence (150+ Connection)

Symptoms Noticed: ____

Food/Supplements: ____

Daily Vitality Log

The Morning Baseline

Date: _____/_____/_______   Date of Cycle: _____/_____/_______

Blood Pressure: ____ / ____

Waking Glucose: _________   Weight: ___________

The PCOS Cycle Tracker

Flow: [ ] Light   [ ] Med   [ ] Heavy   [ ] Spotting

Ovulation Test: [ ] Positive   [ ] Negative

Cervical Fluid Type: ________   Basal Body Temp: _______

Grooming Log

[ ] Shave   [ ] Wax   [ ] Thread   [ ] Laser

Intensity Scale: 1   2   3   4   5

Daily Habits & Triggers

Movement Goal: [ ] Done!

Mood: 1   2   3   4   5   Energy: 1   2   3   4   5

Caffeine: Alcohol:

The Evidence (150+ Connection)

Symptoms Noticed: ____

Food/Supplements: ____

Daily Vitality Log

The Morning Baseline

Date: _____/_____/_______   Date of Cycle: _____/_____/________

Blood Pressure: ____ / ____

Waking Glucose: __________   Weight: ____________

The PCOS Cycle Tracker

Flow: [ ] Light   [ ] Med   [ ] Heavy   [ ] Spotting

Ovulation Test: [ ] Positive   [ ] Negative

Cervical Fluid Type: _________   Basal Body Temp: _______

Grooming Log

[ ] Shave   [ ] Wax   [ ] Thread   [ ] Laser

Intensity Scale: 1   2   3   4   5

Daily Habits & Triggers

Movement Goal: [ ] Done!

Mood: 1   2   3   4   5   Energy: 1   2   3   4   5

Caffeine: Alcohol:

The Evidence (150+ Connection)

Symptoms Noticed: ____

Food/Supplements: ____

Daily Vitality Log

The Morning Baseline

Date: _____/______/________   Date of Cycle: _____/______/________

Blood Pressure: ____ / ____

Waking Glucose: __________   Weight: ____________

The PCOS Cycle Tracker

Flow: [ ] Light   [ ] Med   [ ] Heavy   [ ] Spotting

Ovulation Test: [ ] Positive   [ ] Negative

Cervical Fluid Type: _________   Basal Body Temp: ________

Grooming Log

[ ] Shave   [ ] Wax   [ ] Thread   [ ] Laser

Intensity Scale: 1   2   3   4   5

Daily Habits & Triggers

Movement Goal: [ ] Done!

Mood: 1   2   3   4   5   Energy: 1   2   3   4   5

Caffeine: Alcohol:

The Evidence (150+ Connection)

Symptoms Noticed: ____

Food/Supplements: ____

Daily Vitality Log

The Morning Baseline

Date: _____/_____/_______   Date of Cycle: _____/_____/________

Blood Pressure: _____ / _____

Waking Glucose: ___________   Weight: ____________

The PCOS Cycle Tracker

Flow: [ ] Light   [ ] Med   [ ] Heavy   [ ] Spotting

Ovulation Test: [ ] Positive   [ ] Negative

Cervical Fluid Type: _________   Basal Body Temp: ________

Grooming Log

[ ] Shave   [ ] Wax   [ ] Thread   [ ] Laser

Intensity Scale: 1   2   3   4   5

Daily Habits & Triggers

Movement Goal: [ ] Done!

Mood: 1   2   3   4   5   Energy: 1   2   3   4   5

Caffeine: Alcohol:

The Evidence (150+ Connection)

Symptoms Noticed: ____

Food/Supplements: ____

Daily Vitality Log

The Morning Baseline

Date: _____/_____/_______   Date of Cycle: _____/_____/________

Blood Pressure: _____ / _____

Waking Glucose: __________   Weight: ___________

The PCOS Cycle Tracker

Flow: [ ] Light   [ ] Med   [ ] Heavy   [ ] Spotting

Ovulation Test: [ ] Positive   [ ] Negative

Cervical Fluid Type: _________   Basal Body Temp: ________

Grooming Log

[ ] Shave   [ ] Wax   [ ] Thread   [ ] Laser

Intensity Scale: 1   2   3   4   5

Daily Habits & Triggers

Movement Goal: [ ] Done!

Mood: 1   2   3   4   5   Energy: 1   2   3   4   5

Caffeine: Alcohol:

The Evidence (150+ Connection)

Symptoms Noticed: ____

Food/Supplements: ____

Daily Vitality Log

The Morning Baseline

Date: _____/______/________   Date of Cycle: _____/______/________

Blood Pressure: ____ / ____

Waking Glucose: __________   Weight: ___________

The PCOS Cycle Tracker

Flow: [ ] Light   [ ] Med   [ ] Heavy   [ ] Spotting

Ovulation Test: [ ] Positive   [ ] Negative

Cervical Fluid Type: _________   Basal Body Temp: ________

Grooming Log

[ ] Shave   [ ] Wax   [ ] Thread   [ ] Laser

Intensity Scale: 1   2   3   4   5

Daily Habits & Triggers

Movement Goal: [ ] Done!

Mood: 1   2   3   4   5   Energy: 1   2   3   4   5

Caffeine: Alcohol:

The Evidence (150+ Connection)

Symptoms Noticed: ____

Food/Supplements: ____

Daily Vitality Log

The Morning Baseline

Date: _____/_____/_______   Date of Cycle: _____/_____/________

Blood Pressure: ____ / ____

Waking Glucose: __________   Weight: ___________

The PCOS Cycle Tracker

Flow: [ ] Light   [ ] Med   [ ] Heavy   [ ] Spotting

Ovulation Test: [ ] Positive   [ ] Negative

Cervical Fluid Type: _________   Basal Body Temp: _______

Grooming Log

[ ] Shave   [ ] Wax   [ ] Thread   [ ] Laser

Intensity Scale: 1   2   3   4   5

Daily Habits & Triggers

Movement Goal: [ ] Done!

Mood: 1   2   3   4   5   Energy: 1   2   3   4   5

Caffeine: Alcohol:

The Evidence (150+ Connection)

Symptoms Noticed: ____

Food/Supplements: ____

Daily Vitality Log

The Morning Baseline

Date: _____/_____/_______   Date of Cycle: _____/_____/_______

❤ Blood Pressure: _____ / _____

Waking Glucose: __________   Weight: ____________

The PCOS Cycle Tracker

Flow: [ ] Light   [ ] Med   [ ] Heavy   [ ] Spotting

Ovulation Test: [ ] Positive   [ ] Negative

Cervical Fluid Type: _________   Basal Body Temp: _______

Grooming Log

[ ] Shave   [ ] Wax   [ ] Thread   [ ] Laser

Intensity Scale: 1   2   3   4   5

Daily Habits & Triggers

Movement Goal: [ ] Done!

Mood: 1   2   3   4   5   Energy: 1   2   3   4   5

Caffeine: Alcohol:

The Evidence (150+ Connection)

Symptoms Noticed: ____

Food/Supplements: ____

Daily Vitality Log

The Morning Baseline

Date: _____/_____/______   Date of Cycle: _____/_____/________

Blood Pressure: ____ / ____

Waking Glucose: __________   Weight: ___________

The PCOS Cycle Tracker

Flow: [ ] Light   [ ] Med   [ ] Heavy   [ ] Spotting

Ovulation Test: [ ] Positive   [ ] Negative

Cervical Fluid Type: _________   Basal Body Temp: _______

Grooming Log

[ ] Shave   [ ] Wax   [ ] Thread   [ ] Laser

Intensity Scale: 1   2   3   4   5

Daily Habits & Triggers

Movement Goal: [ ] Done!

Mood: 1   2   3   4   5   Energy: 1   2   3   4   5

Caffeine: Alcohol:

The Evidence (150+ Connection)

Symptoms Noticed: ____

Food/Supplements: ____

Daily Vitality Log

The Morning Baseline

Date: _____/_____/______   Date of Cycle: _____/_____/_______

Blood Pressure: _____/_____

Waking Glucose: __________   Weight: ___________

The PCOS Cycle Tracker

Flow: [ ] Light   [ ] Med   [ ] Heavy   [ ] Spotting

Ovulation Test: [ ] Positive   [ ] Negative

Cervical Fluid Type: _________   Basal Body Temp: ________

Grooming Log

[ ] Shave   [ ] Wax   [ ] Thread   [ ] Laser

Intensity Scale: 1   2   3   4   5

Daily Habits & Triggers

Movement Goal: [ ] Done!

Mood: 1   2   3   4   5   Energy: 1   2   3   4   5

Caffeine: Alcohol:

The Evidence (150+ Connection)

Symptoms Noticed: ____

Food/Supplements: ____

Daily Vitality Log

The Morning Baseline

Date: _____/______/_______   Date of Cycle: _____/______/________

Blood Pressure: ____ / ____

Waking Glucose: __________   Weight: ____________

The PCOS Cycle Tracker

Flow: [ ] Light   [ ] Med   [ ] Heavy   [ ] Spotting

Ovulation Test: [ ] Positive   [ ] Negative

Cervical Fluid Type: _________   Basal Body Temp: ________

Grooming Log

[ ] Shave   [ ] Wax   [ ] Thread   [ ] Laser

Intensity Scale: 1   2   3   4   5

Daily Habits & Triggers

Movement Goal: [ ] Done!

Mood: 1   2   3   4   5   Energy: 1   2   3   4   5

Caffeine: ☕ ☕ ☕   Alcohol: 🍷 🍷 🍷

The Evidence (150+ Connection)

Symptoms Noticed: ____

Food/Supplements: ____

Daily Vitality Log

The Morning Baseline

Date: _____/______/________   Date of Cycle: ______/______/________

Blood Pressure: _____ / _____

Waking Glucose: ___________   Weight: _____________

The PCOS Cycle Tracker

Flow: [ ] Light   [ ] Med   [ ] Heavy   [ ] Spotting

Ovulation Test: [ ] Positive   [ ] Negative

Cervical Fluid Type: _________   Basal Body Temp: ________

Grooming Log

[ ] Shave   [ ] Wax   [ ] Thread   [ ] Laser

Intensity Scale: 1   2   3   4   5

Daily Habits & Triggers

Movement Goal: [ ] Done!

Mood: 1   2   3   4   5   Energy: 1   2   3   4   5

Caffeine: Alcohol:

The Evidence (150+ Connection)

Symptoms Noticed: ____

Food/Supplements: ____

Daily Vitality Log

The Morning Baseline

Date: _____/______/_______   Date of Cycle: _____/______/________

Blood Pressure: ____ / ____

Waking Glucose: __________   Weight: ____________

The PCOS Cycle Tracker

Flow: [ ] Light   [ ] Med   [ ] Heavy   [ ] Spotting

Ovulation Test: [ ] Positive   [ ] Negative

Cervical Fluid Type: _________   Basal Body Temp: _______

Grooming Log

[ ] Shave   [ ] Wax   [ ] Thread   [ ] Laser

Intensity Scale: 1   2   3   4   5

Daily Habits & Triggers

Movement Goal: [ ] Done!

Mood: 1   2   3   4   5   Energy: 1   2   3   4   5

Caffeine: Alcohol:

The Evidence (150+ Connection)

Symptoms Noticed: ____

Food/Supplements: ____

Daily Vitality Log

The Morning Baseline

Date: _____/_____/________   Date of Cycle: _____/_____/________

Blood Pressure: _____ / _____

Waking Glucose: ___________   Weight: ___________

The PCOS Cycle Tracker

Flow: [ ] Light   [ ] Med   [ ] Heavy   [ ] Spotting

Ovulation Test: [ ] Positive   [ ] Negative

Cervical Fluid Type: _________   Basal Body Temp: ________

Grooming Log

[ ] Shave   [ ] Wax   [ ] Thread   [ ] Laser

Intensity Scale: 1   2   3   4   5

Daily Habits & Triggers

Movement Goal: [ ] Done!

Mood: 1   2   3   4   5   Energy: 1   2   3   4   5

Caffeine: Alcohol:

The Evidence (150+ Connection)

Symptoms Noticed: ____

Food/Supplements: ____

Daily Vitality Log

The Morning Baseline

Date: _____/_____/______   Date of Cycle: _____/_____/_______

Blood Pressure: ____ / ____

Waking Glucose: __________   Weight: ___________

The PCOS Cycle Tracker

Flow: [ ] Light   [ ] Med   [ ] Heavy   [ ] Spotting

Ovulation Test: [ ] Positive   [ ] Negative

Cervical Fluid Type: __________   Basal Body Temp: ________

Grooming Log

[ ] Shave   [ ] Wax   [ ] Thread   [ ] Laser

Intensity Scale: 1   2   3   4   5

Daily Habits & Triggers

Movement Goal: [ ] Done!

Mood: 1   2   3   4   5   Energy: 1   2   3   4   5

Caffeine: Alcohol:

The Evidence (150+ Connection)

Symptoms Noticed: ____

Food/Supplements: ____

Daily Vitality Log

The Morning Baseline

Date: _____/_____/_______   Date of Cycle: _____/_____/________

Blood Pressure: _____ / _____

Waking Glucose: ___________   Weight: ____________

The PCOS Cycle Tracker

Flow: [ ] Light   [ ] Med   [ ] Heavy   [ ] Spotting

Ovulation Test: [ ] Positive   [ ] Negative

Cervical Fluid Type: _________   Basal Body Temp: ________

Grooming Log

[ ] Shave   [ ] Wax   [ ] Thread   [ ] Laser

Intensity Scale: 1   2   3   4   5

Daily Habits & Triggers

Movement Goal: [ ] Done!

Mood: 1   2   3   4   5   Energy: 1   2   3   4   5

Caffeine: Alcohol:

The Evidence (150+ Connection)

Symptoms Noticed: ____

Food/Supplements: ____

Daily Vitality Log

The Morning Baseline

Date: _____/______/_______   Date of Cycle: ____`/______/________

Blood Pressure: ____ / ____

Waking Glucose: __________   Weight: ___________

The PCOS Cycle Tracker

Flow: [ ] Light   [ ] Med   [ ] Heavy   [ ] Spotting

Ovulation Test: [ ] Positive   [ ] Negative

Cervical Fluid Type: _________   Basal Body Temp: ________

Grooming Log

[ ] Shave   [ ] Wax   [ ] Thread   [ ] Laser

Intensity Scale: 1   2   3   4   5

Daily Habits & Triggers

Movement Goal: [ ] Done!

Mood: 1   2   3   4   5   Energy: 1   2   3   4   5

Caffeine: Alcohol:

The Evidence (150+ Connection)

Symptoms Noticed: ____

Food/Supplements: ____

Daily Vitality Log

The Morning Baseline

Date: _____/______/________   Date of Cycle: ______/______/__________

♥ Blood Pressure: _____ / _____

Waking Glucose: ___________   Weight: ______________

The PCOS Cycle Tracker

Flow: [ ] Light   [ ] Med   [ ] Heavy   [ ] Spotting

Ovulation Test: [ ] Positive   [ ] Negative

Cervical Fluid Type: __________   Basal Body Temp: ________

Grooming Log

[ ] Shave   [ ] Wax   [ ] Thread   [ ] Laser

Intensity Scale: 1   2   3   4   5

Daily Habits & Triggers

Movement Goal: [ ] Done!

Mood: 1   2   3   4   5   Energy: 1   2   3   4   5

Caffeine: Alcohol:

The Evidence (150+ Connection)

Symptoms Noticed: ____

Food/Supplements: ____

Daily Vitality Log

The Morning Baseline

Date: _____/_____/_______   Date of Cycle: _____/_____/________

Blood Pressure: ____ / ____

Waking Glucose: __________   Weight: ___________

The PCOS Cycle Tracker

Flow: [ ] Light   [ ] Med   [ ] Heavy   [ ] Spotting

Ovulation Test: [ ] Positive   [ ] Negative

Cervical Fluid Type: _________   Basal Body Temp: _______

Grooming Log

[ ] Shave   [ ] Wax   [ ] Thread   [ ] Laser

Intensity Scale: 1   2   3   4   5

Daily Habits & Triggers

Movement Goal: [ ] Done!

Mood: 1   2   3   4   5   Energy: 1   2   3   4   5

Caffeine: Alcohol:

The Evidence (150+ Connection)

Symptoms Noticed: ____

Food/Supplements: ____

Daily Vitality Log

The Morning Baseline

Date: _____/_____/_______   Date of Cycle: _____/_____/________

♥ Blood Pressure: ____ / ____

Waking Glucose: __________   Weight: ___________

The PCOS Cycle Tracker

Flow: [ ] Light   [ ] Med   [ ] Heavy   [ ] Spotting

Ovulation Test: [ ] Positive   [ ] Negative

Cervical Fluid Type: ________   Basal Body Temp: _______

Grooming Log

[ ] Shave   [ ] Wax   [ ] Thread   [ ] Laser

Intensity Scale: 1   2   3   4   5

Daily Habits & Triggers

Movement Goal: [ ] Done!

Mood: 1   2   3   4   5   Energy: 1   2   3   4   5

Caffeine: Alcohol:

The Evidence (150+ Connection)

Symptoms Noticed: ____

Food/Supplements: ____

Daily Vitality Log

The Morning Baseline

Date: _____/______/________   Date of Cycle: _____/______/________

Blood Pressure: ____ / ____

Waking Glucose: __________   Weight: ____________

The PCOS Cycle Tracker

Flow: [ ] Light   [ ] Med   [ ] Heavy   [ ] Spotting

Ovulation Test: [ ] Positive   [ ] Negative

Cervical Fluid Type: _________   Basal Body Temp: ________

Grooming Log

[ ] Shave   [ ] Wax   [ ] Thread   [ ] Laser

Intensity Scale: 1   2   3   4   5

Daily Habits & Triggers

Movement Goal: [ ] Done!

Mood: 1   2   3   4   5   Energy: 1   2   3   4   5

Caffeine: Alcohol:

The Evidence (150+ Connection)

Symptoms Noticed: ____

Food/Supplements: ____

Daily Vitality Log

The Morning Baseline

Date: _____/_____/______   Date of Cycle: _____/_____/_______

❤ Blood Pressure: _____ / _____

Waking Glucose: __________   Weight: ___________

The PCOS Cycle Tracker

Flow: [ ] Light   [ ] Med   [ ] Heavy   [ ] Spotting

Ovulation Test: [ ] Positive   [ ] Negative

Cervical Fluid Type: _________   Basal Body Temp: _______

Grooming Log

[ ] Shave   [ ] Wax   [ ] Thread   [ ] Laser

Intensity Scale: 1   2   3   4   5

Daily Habits & Triggers

Movement Goal: [ ] Done!

Mood: 1   2   3   4   5   Energy: 1   2   3   4   5

Caffeine: Alcohol:

The Evidence (150+ Connection)

Symptoms Noticed: ____

Food/Supplements: ____

Daily Vitality Log

The Morning Baseline

Date: _____/______/________   Date of Cycle: _____/______/________

Blood Pressure: _____ / _____

Waking Glucose: ___________   Weight: ____________

The PCOS Cycle Tracker

Flow: [ ] Light   [ ] Med   [ ] Heavy   [ ] Spotting

Ovulation Test: [ ] Positive   [ ] Negative

Cervical Fluid Type: _________   Basal Body Temp: ________

Grooming Log

[ ] Shave   [ ] Wax   [ ] Thread   [ ] Laser

Intensity Scale: 1   2   3   4   5

Daily Habits & Triggers

Movement Goal: [ ] Done!

Mood: 1   2   3   4   5   Energy: 1   2   3   4   5

Caffeine: Alcohol:

The Evidence (150+ Connection)

Symptoms Noticed: ____

Food/Supplements: ____

The 90-Day Reflection & Report

Starting Weight: ___________   Final Weight: ___________

Avg. Morning Glucose (Month 1): _____________

Avg. Morning Glucose (Month 3): _____________

Blood Pressure Trend: ____

Total Cycles Tracked: _________ Days with Positive Ovulation: _________

The "Grooming Glow" Result: (e.g., Shaving frequency went from 1

day to 4 days): _________________

Top 3 Signals that Improved:

1.____

2.____

3.____

Write your top 3 concerns or questions for your next specialist
visit here:

1.____

2.____

3.____

The Authority & Strategy Page

Evidence-Based Tracking: The symptoms listed in this protocol are clinically linked to Androgen Excess, Insulin Resistance, and Chronic Inflammation.

The "Signal" Philosophy: Research shows that PCOS is a multi-system metabolic disorder, meaning "random glitches" like skin tags, dry eyes, and anxiety are often biometric signals of hormonal shifts.

Consult Your Specialist: Always share these patterns with your Endocrinologist or OBGYN to refine your personal medical blueprint.

Primary Goals for Phase 2:

1.____

2.____

3. ____

Non-Scale Victory (NSV) to Chase:

____

One Habit I'm Keeping:

____

____

Scientific References & Final Protocol Disclaimer

- **The 150+ Connection:** *The symptoms and conditions listed within this protocol are based on established clinical overlaps between Polycystic Ovary Syndrome (PCOS), Insulin Resistance, and Androgen Excess.*
- **Biometric Standards:** *The tracking of Waking Glucose and Blood Pressure follows metabolic health monitoring guidelines supported by the American Diabetes Association (ADA).*
- **Hirsutism Intelligence:** *Tracking hair growth frequency (Grooming Log) is a recognized method for monitoring the physical markers of hormonal shifts.*

- **PCOS Awareness Association (PCOSAA):** For the comprehensive mapping of associated metabolic and systemic conditions.
- **The Endocrine Society:** Clinical guidelines regarding the management of PCOS-related symptoms and insulin strategy.
- **Womenshealth.gov (Office on Women's Health):** For peer-reviewed education on reproductive health and hormonal balance.

Notes, Breakthroughs & Future Intelligence

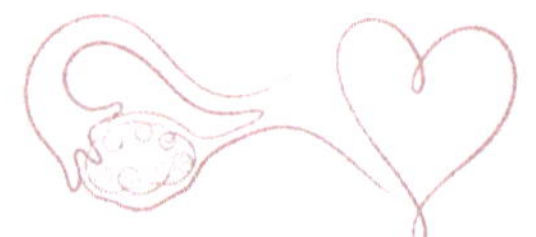

Notes, Breakthroughs & Future Intelligence

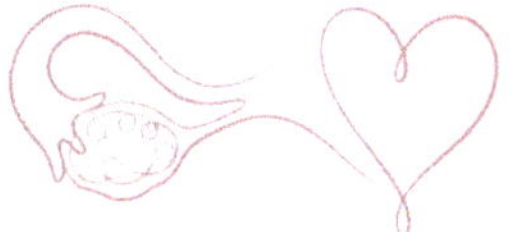

Meet the Visionary & Aivonax

The Aivonax Story: *"As a tech girl with a small business, I realized Aivonax had to become more than just building websites. It had to be about building intelligent operations for our lives. This logbook is our first step into high-impact digital and physical products—turning your 150+ 'glitches' into a data-driven map so you can take your strength back."*

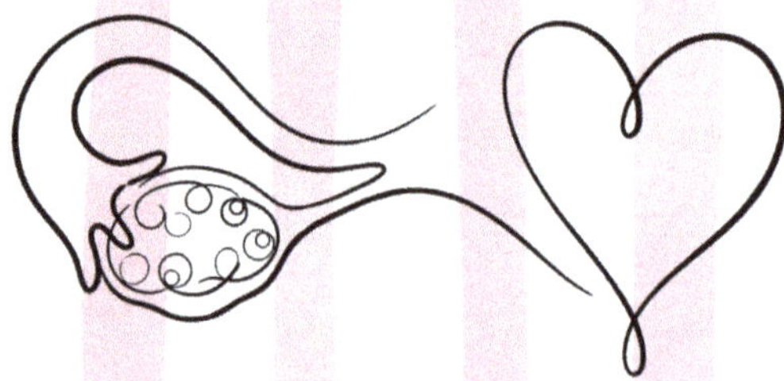

The Team:

Lead Author & Visionary: Angela Hayes — A Roseville-based entrepreneur and IT specialist who transitioned from troubleshooting servers to troubleshooting the PCOS journey.

Strategic Operations: An intelligent operations company focused on tech-forward digital products and system-driven wellness.

Design & Layout: The Aivonax Creative Team.

Connect with the Operation
- Official Website: www.aivonax.com
- The Digital Hub: linktr.ee/angytheceo

www.ingramcontent.com/pod-product-compliance
Lightning Source LLC
Chambersburg PA
CBHW040123150726
48005CB00015B/2338